As you read this book you will be able to find the answers to many questions about yourself and the way you do things. This book is based on the popular 'Me and My Body' exhibition at **EUREKA! The Museum for Children** in Halifax. **EUREKA!** is the first museum in Great Britain designed especially for children. The Museum's exhibitions use an exciting new approach, placing the child at the centre of learning, and the book has been designed to bring the best of the exhibition into your home or classroom.

The book is full of activities and information. It offers plenty of talking points for children and adults and shows how learning together can be fun. The book will appeal to the child in us all.

EUREKA! The Museum for Children 1994

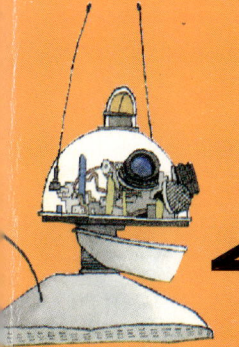

Help me to find out all there is to know about yourselves - your outsides and your insides, your feelings and your dreams.

ACKNOWLEDGEMENTS

Riverswift would like to thank the following
for their kind co-operation in the making of this book:

Boots the Chemists; James Gale & Co; Early Learning Centre; Olympus Sports;
Chamberlain's Cycles, Kentish Town; Peter Seamer at Educational & Scientific Products
Ltd; the children of Macaulay School, Balham and their families; Alex Bartel, Science
Photo Library for the photograph on p.26
Models from EUREKA! and exhibition design by Imagination Ltd, McAndroids and Satoshi Kitamura

Photography by Katie Vandyck and Charles Best
Design by Mandy Sherliker

First published 1994

1 3 5 7 9 10 8 6 4 2

Text © Stephen Webster 1994
Illustrations © Satoshi Kitamura 1994
Stephen Webster and Satoshi Kitamura have asserted their
right under the Copyright, Designs and Patents Act, 1988
to be identified as the author and illustrator of this work.

First published in the United Kingdom in 1994 by
Riverswift
Random House, 20 Vauxhall Bridge Road, London SW1V 2SA

Random House Australia (Pty) Limited
20 Alfred Street, Milsons Point, Sydney,
New South Wales 2061, Australia

Random House New Zealand Limited
18 Poland Road, Glenfield
Auckland 10, New Zealand

Random House South Africa (Pty) Limited
PO Box 337, Bergvlei, South Africa

Random House UK Limited Reg. No. 954009

The EUREKA! series of books is based on the displays at
EUREKA! The Museum for Children, Discovery Road, Halifax,
Yorkshire, England, HX1 2NE. Tel: 0422 330069

A CIP Catalogue record for this book is
available from the British Library

ISBN 1 898304 41 6
Printed in Hong Kong

Me and My Body

A EUREKA!™ Book

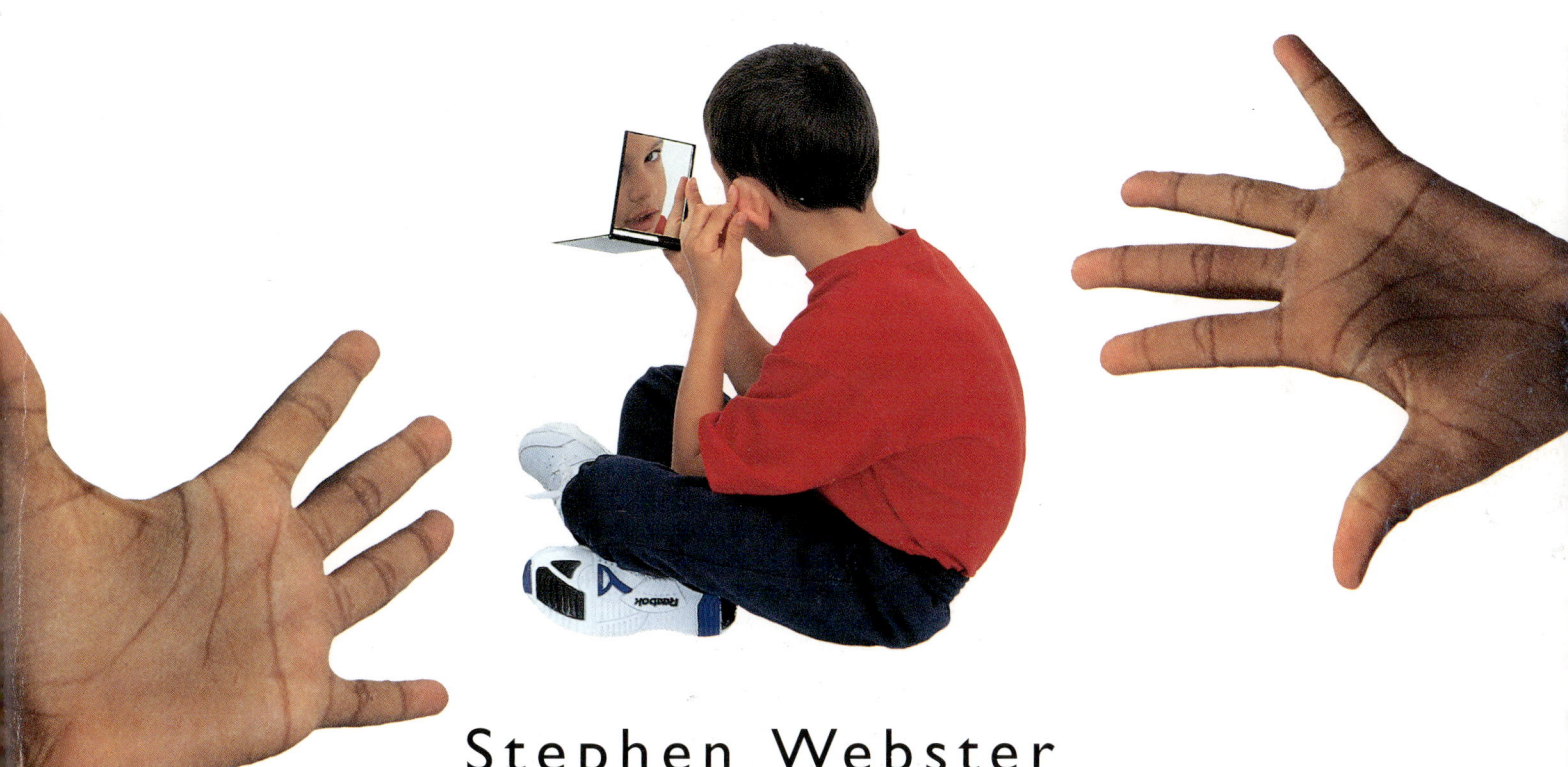

Stephen Webster

Illustrations by Satoshi Kitamura

RIVERSWIFT
LONDON

ME AND MY BODY

Who am I?

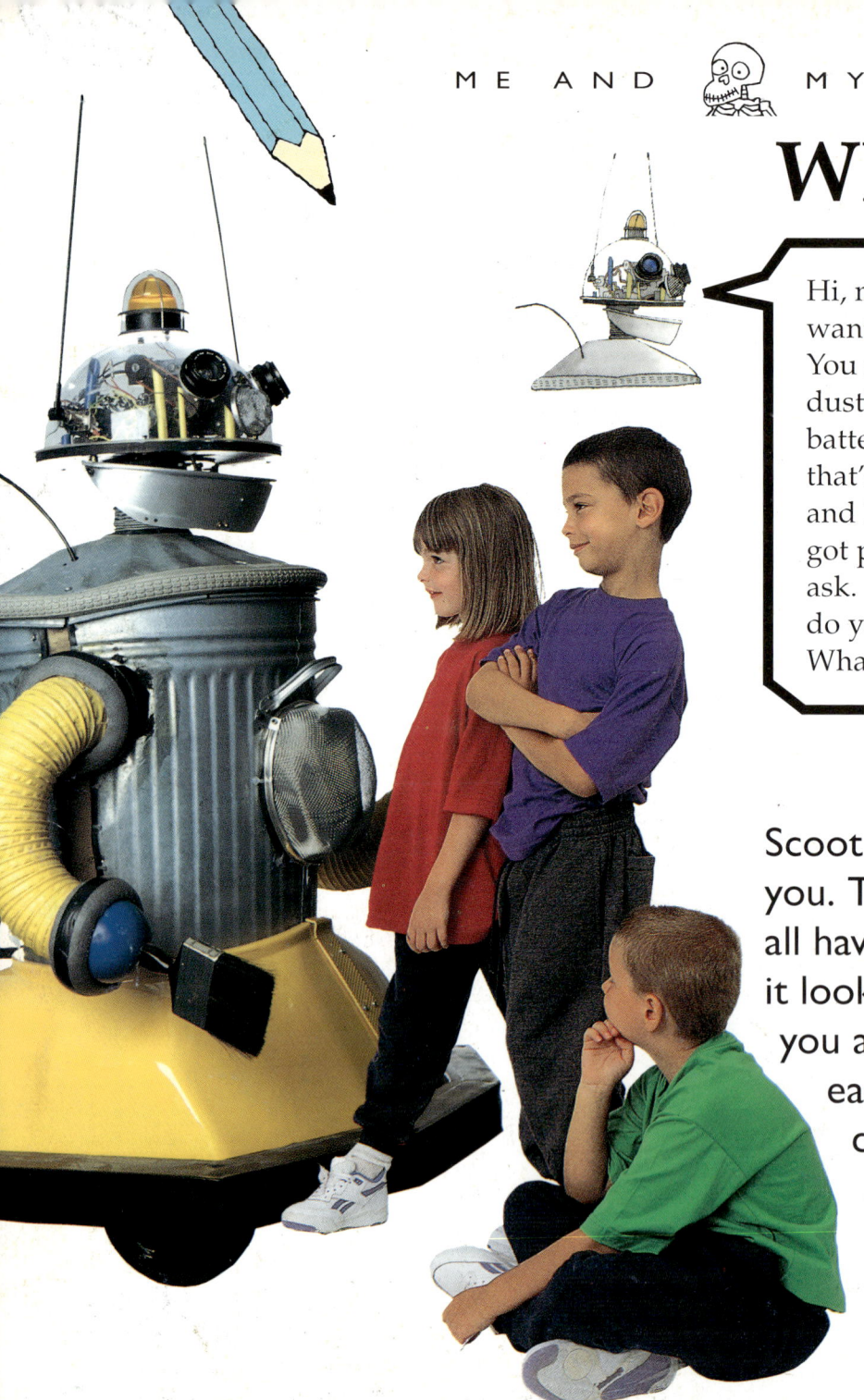

Hi, my name is Scoot! I'm a robot and I want to find out about you and your body. You see, I'm made very simply. An old dustbin, some plastic, a lot of wire, two batteries, and some other bits and pieces - that's me! I can't do things like you can and I don't feel things, either. But I've got plenty of questions to ask. Who are you? What do you like doing? What's inside you?

Scoot wants to find out about you. The robot can see that you all have similar bodies, but when it looks more closely it sees that you are all quite different from each other. You have different coloured hair and eyes and skin. You all tell Scoot that you have quite different likes and dislikes, too.

ME AND MY BODY

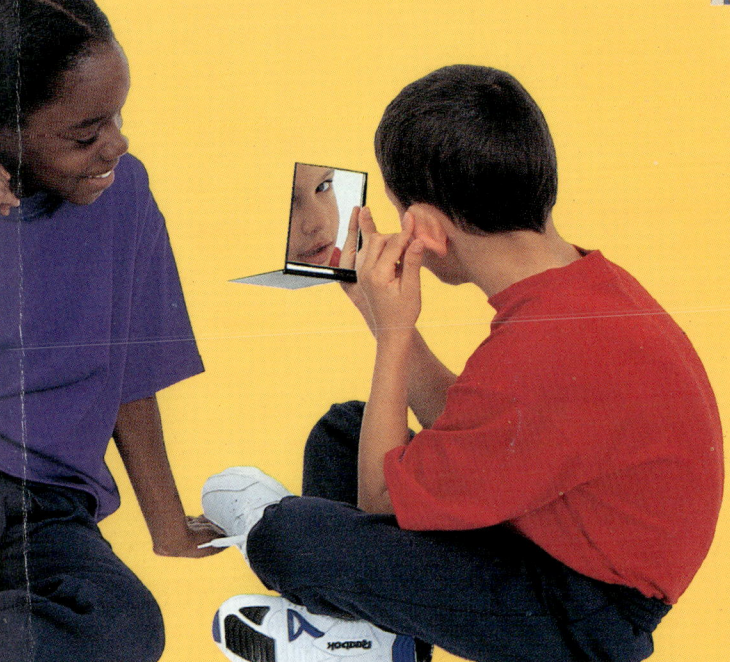

Make some lists:
Which games do you like best?
What is your favourite colour?
Who are your friends?
Who are the people in your family?
What are your favourite books, films and TV programmes?

Scoot investigates

Note it down
Find a large notebook to record your investigations. This can be your special book. Put your name and age on the front.

Write
Look in a mirror and write a description of your face. Read it to someone else. Can they recognise you from your description?

Draw
Make a picture of the outline of your body on a large piece of paper. Draw what you think is inside your body. Don't forget your brain!

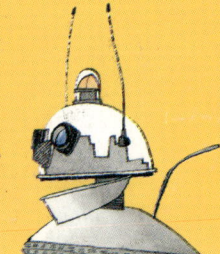

I've started to learn a bit about you. In some ways children are the same, but in others they are all different.

ME AND MY BODY

I'm like this

> I've noticed something else important. Children are all different sizes. You don't even wear the same-sized shoes. I need to have your measurements to help me understand the human body. How tall are you? How long are your legs?

Your body is getting bigger all the time. You won't stop growing until you are between the ages of sixteen and nineteen.

Once you are grown up you won't get any taller. Even children of the same age have different body measurements. In every class or group of friends there is a variety of heights and weights. There isn't really a 'normal' body. You all grow at your own speed.

Your height and your weight can change quite fast. So can your handspan. So it is interesting to measure these things over several months to see how fast you are growing. You can also keep a record of how far you can jump or how high you can reach.

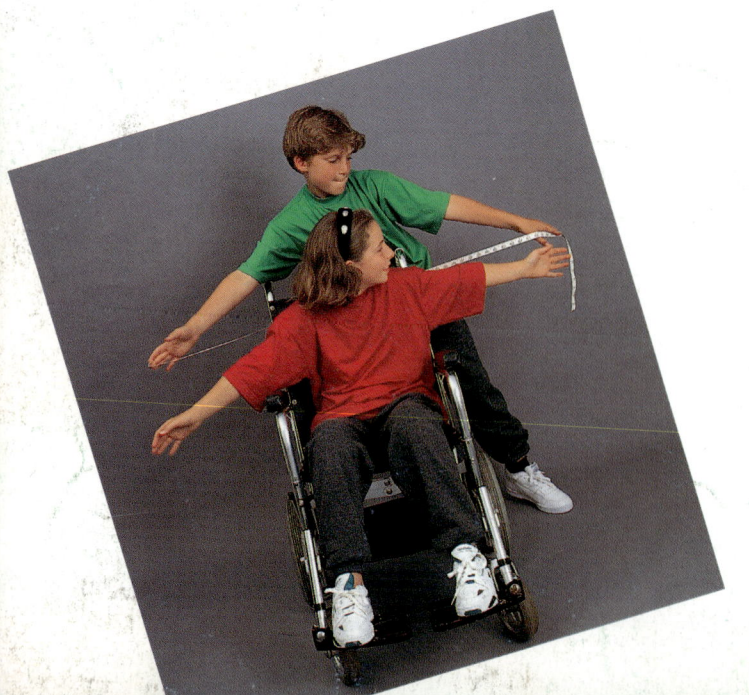
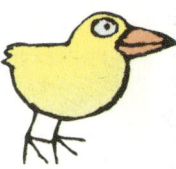
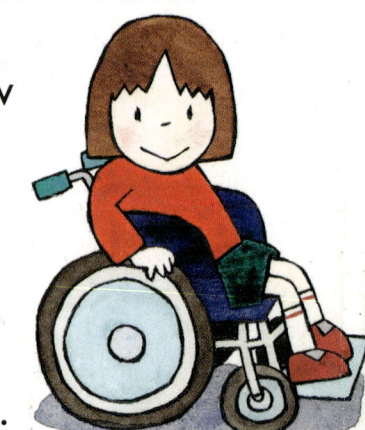

Scoot investigates

Note it down
Make a chart for recording your height and weight and handspan every month for a year. Then fill it in for this month. Here are some other things you could measure and chart:
• The distance round your head
• How far you can stretch with your arms
• How far up you can reach
• The length of your foot
• Your stride

> Now I know this about your bodies: you come in different sizes and you can do all sorts of things. But perhaps I should find out about your feelings too.

My Height
January
February
March
April
May
June
July
August
September
October
November
December

My Weight
January
February
March
April
May
June
July
August
September
October
November
December

ME AND MY BODY

My feelings

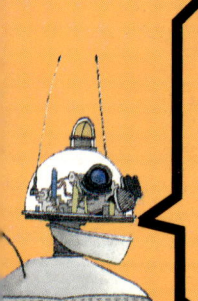

> Now, about me. My problem is that I don't have feelings. How could I? After all, I'm just a machine. You have feelings all the time. So what are they for? Where do you keep them? Do you think I should get some?

Everyone knows the feeling of hunger before a meal. It's the body's way of saying that it needs to eat.

Feelings like sadness, happiness, jealousy and fear are called emotions. They take place in your mind, but you can often show your emotions in your expressions. Most people smile when they are happy! There are a lot of emotions that you feel in other parts of your body too – some people clench their fists when they are angry or get tummy aches when they are nervous. So your body gives you clues to these sorts of feelings as well, and helps you decide what to do next.

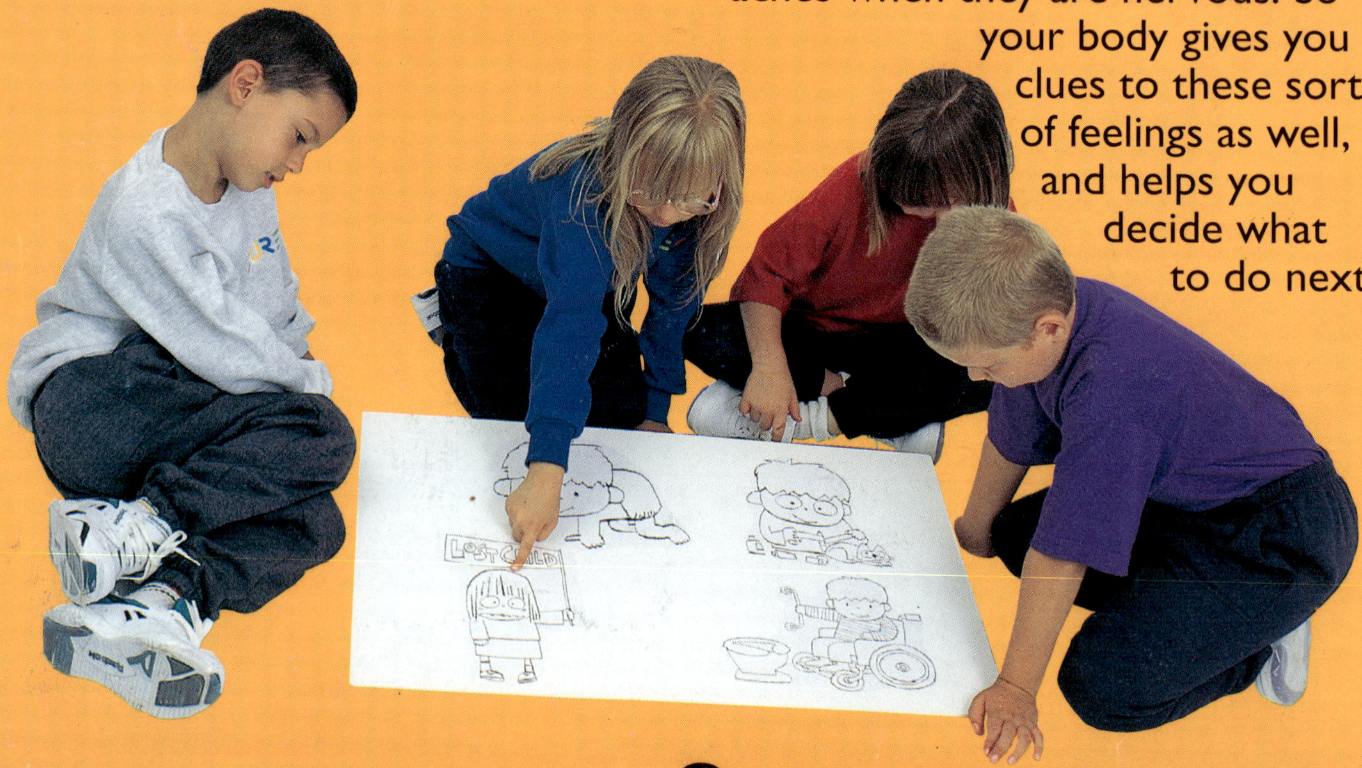

ME AND MY BODY

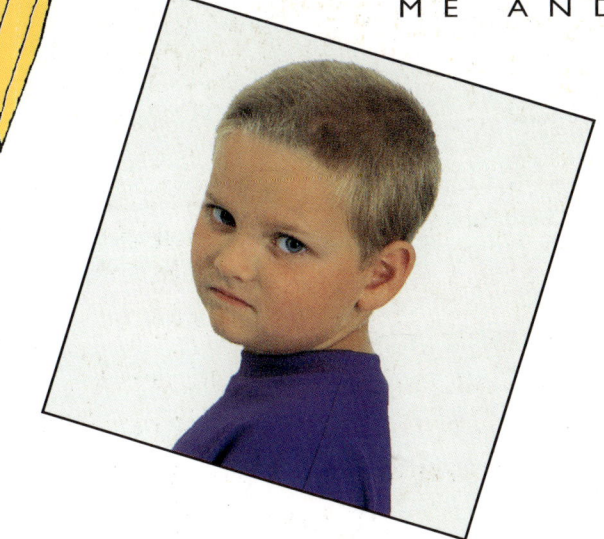

Scoot investigates

Note it down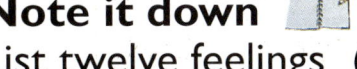
List twelve feelings (like 'happy', 'sad', 'angry') round a circle, like the numbers of a clock. Which word expresses the way you are feeling today?

Imagine the following things happen: You are lost at the shops.

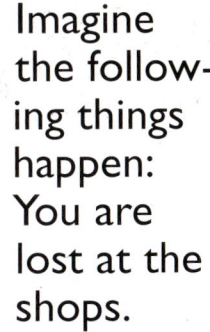

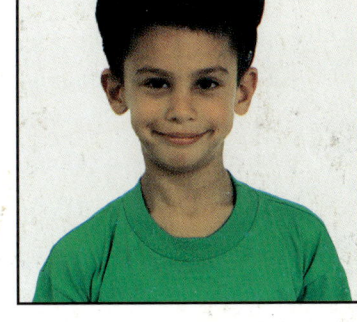

Your mum tells you she is going to have a baby. Your pet is hurt. Your sister wins a prize in a competition. What would you feel about each one?

Write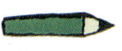
Write a poem which describes how you feel on a good day.

Draw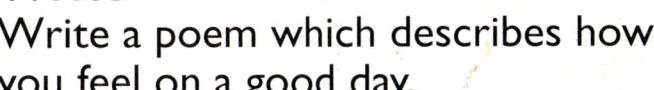
Draw a picture showing someone you know being happy.

Maybe one day I'll learn to have feelings. I wonder what an angry robot would be like? If I had feelings life might be more interesting.

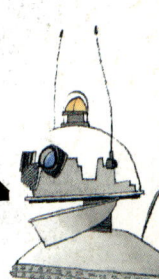

ME AND 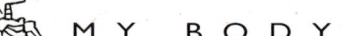 MY BODY

I can do anything

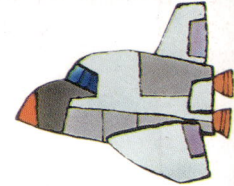

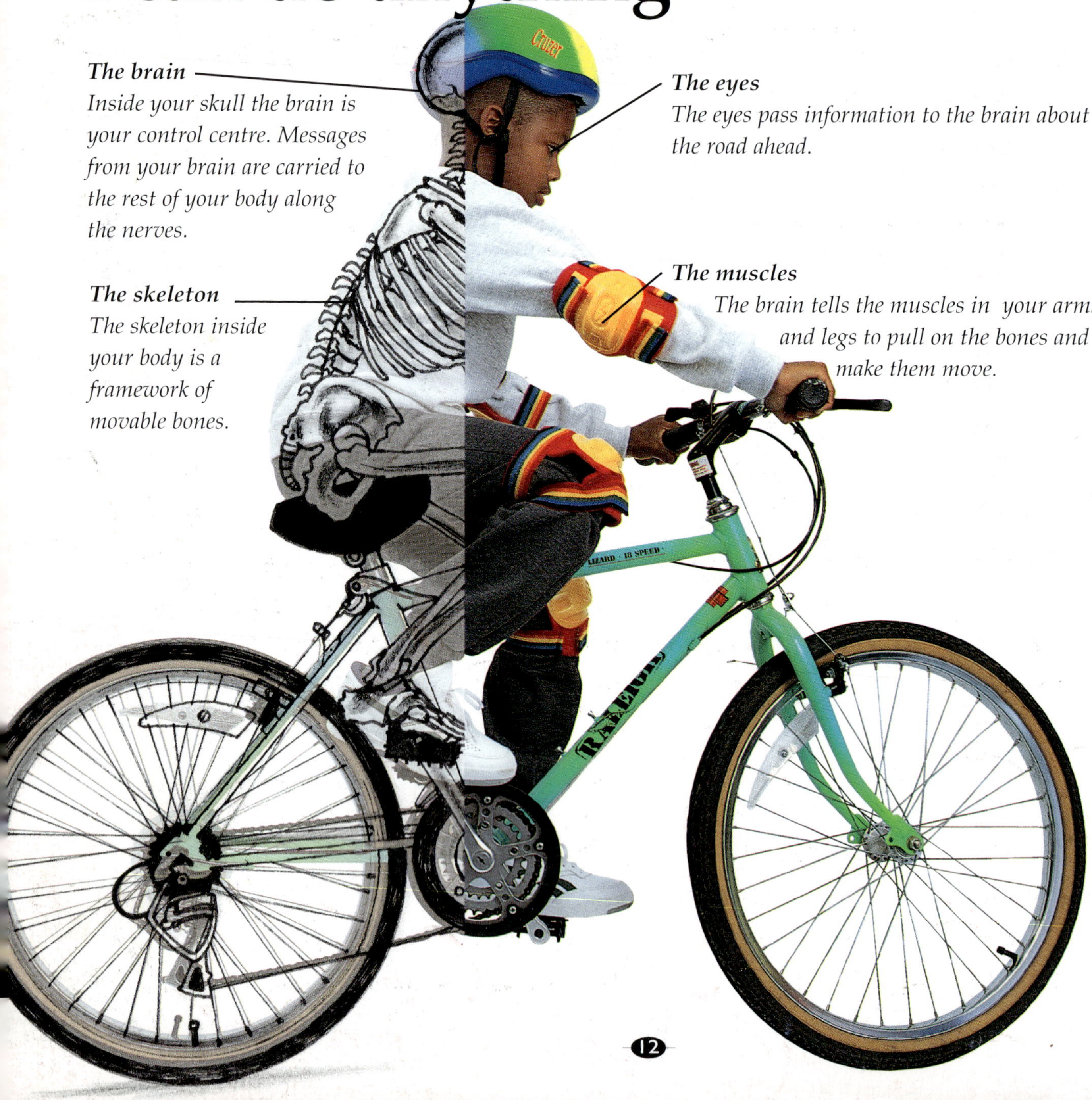

The brain
Inside your skull the brain is your control centre. Messages from your brain are carried to the rest of your body along the nerves.

The skeleton
The skeleton inside your body is a framework of movable bones.

The eyes
The eyes pass information to the brain about the road ahead.

The muscles
The brain tells the muscles in your arms and legs to pull on the bones and make them move.

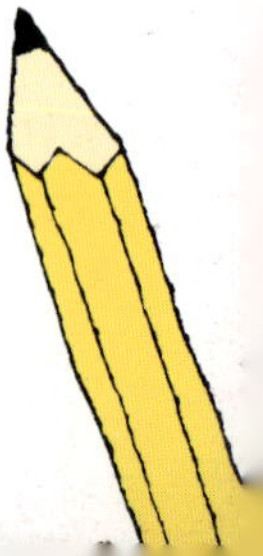

ME AND MY BODY

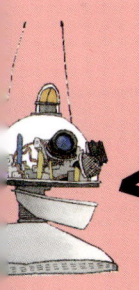

> Riding a bicycle looks easy. You pedal by moving your legs and you change direction by moving your arms. But how does your body know what to do?

Your bones form the framework of your body. Your muscles move your bones. Your brain receives messages from your eyes and ears along the nervous system and controls your movement by sending messages to your muscles. Some disabled people cannot control their movements normally. Probably it is only a tiny part of the body which is not working well. Perhaps the nerves between the brain and muscles are damaged so the messages aren't being received clearly.

Scoot investigates

Experiment

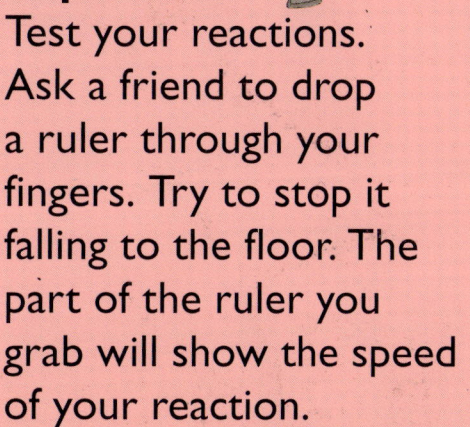

Test your reactions. Ask a friend to drop a ruler through your fingers. Try to stop it falling to the floor. The part of the ruler you grab will show the speed of your reaction.

Test your eyesight. Ask your friend to draw letters on a page, putting the smallest at the bottom. Now stand about two metres away and read out the letters. How far down the page do you get?

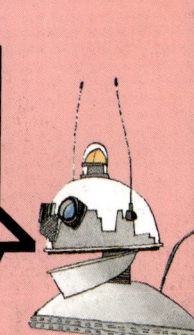

> So movement is controlled by the brain, which sends messages to the muscles. And for the brain to work properly it needs information from your senses. It all sounds very clever!

ME AND MY BODY

What keeps my insides in?

Zebra skin

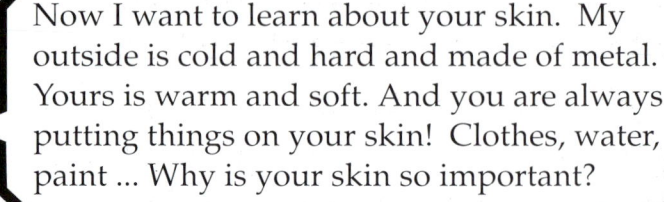

Now I want to learn about your skin. My outside is cold and hard and made of metal. Yours is warm and soft. And you are always putting things on your skin! Clothes, water, paint ... Why is your skin so important?

The skin is the outside part of the body. It covers the muscles, the fat and the blood, keeping them away from harm. One way the skin protects the body is by stopping dirt from getting inside. Cuts and grazes allow germs into the body, which can cause infection.

Your skin grows in layers. The new living layer is at the bottom. It takes six to seven weeks to reach the surface. The surface layer is in fact dead skin that flakes off as it is replaced from below.

ME AND MY BODY

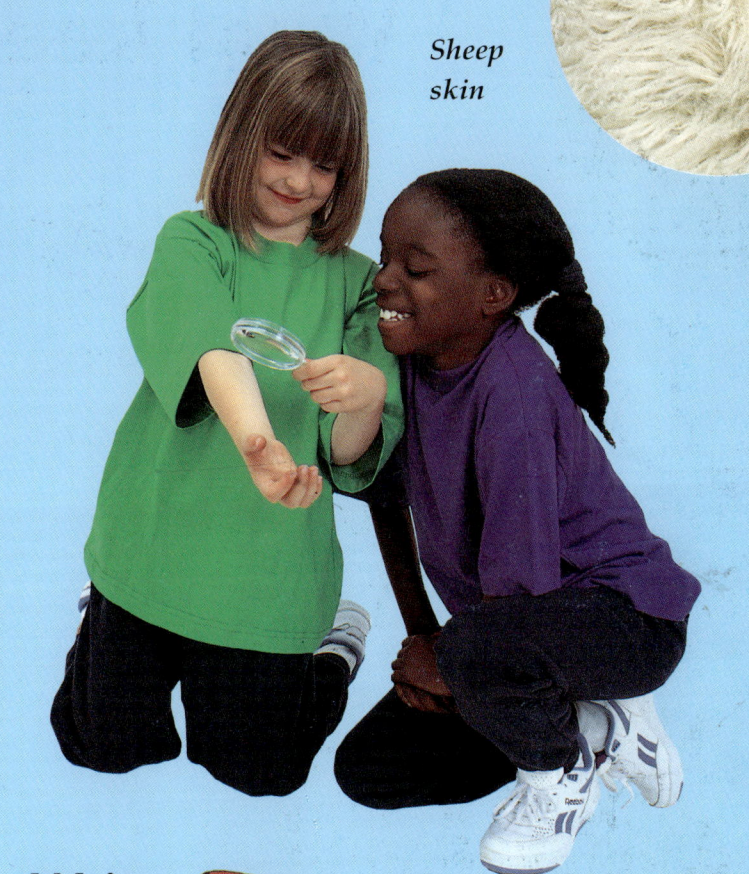

Sheep skin

Skin needs to be looked after, otherwise it cannot do its job. Animal skin is tough or furry, which protects it from damage. Clothing keeps your body warm and also stops the skin from being harmed. You touch and feel things with your skin. Like sight and hearing, touch is one of the senses that send messages to your brain about the world around you.

Scoot investigates

Experiment
Close your eyes, and ask a friend to brush a tissue over the palm of your hand, the back of your hand, your face and your arm. Which bits are the most sensitive? Look at the skin under a magnifying glass. What do you see?

Crocodile skin

Write
Imagine that you wake up one day with a hard metal skin. How might your life change?

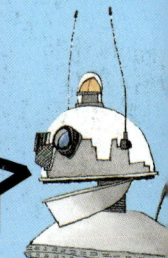

I can see that your skin needs a lot of looking after. But you use it for touching, for protection, even for looking good. Now, I wonder what I can do with my rusty old outside ...

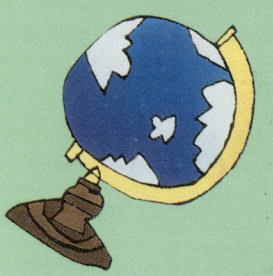

ME AND 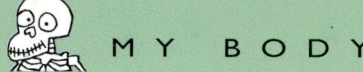 MY BODY

What keeps us going?

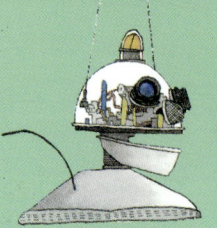

Why do you breathe all the time? You breathe in air, and then you breathe it out. Looks like a waste of time to me.

You breathe because your body needs a gas called oxygen from the air to stay alive. You breathe in air through your nose or mouth. It travels down your windpipe to your lungs. The air contains other gases besides oxygen. In your lungs the oxygen passes into your bloodstream, but the air you breathe out contains the gases (carbon dioxide and water vapour) that your body doesn't need. Part of the brain is always at work, making sure the body keeps breathing all the time. Oxygen is carried to every part of your body in the bloodstream.

ME AND MY BODY

Your heart keeps the blood pumping round your body. When you run around, your muscles work hard and need more oxygen, so your heart and lungs have to work even harder. That is why you pant and take in deep breaths when you have been exercising hard.

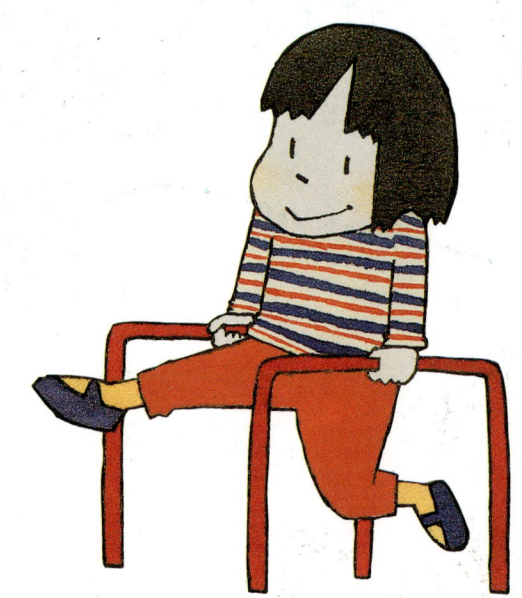

Scoot investigates

Experiment
Measure your pulse rate. You can feel your pulse in your wrist, just below the thumb. Count how many beats you can feel in one minute. Now run on the spot for two minutes and take your pulse again. How many beats did you count this time?

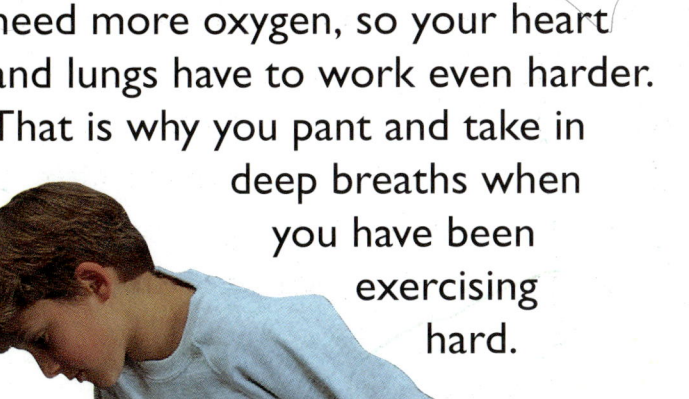

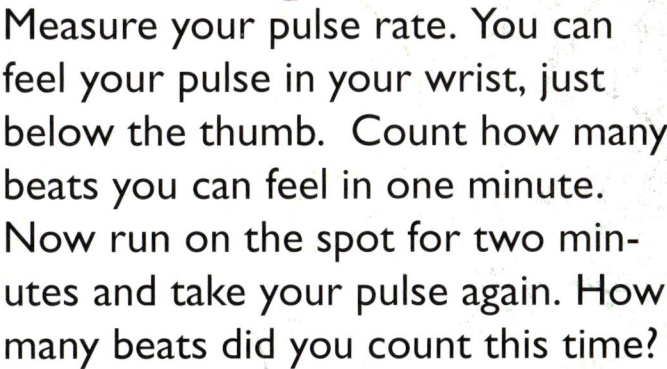

So, your body needs oxygen from the air to work. I wonder what else you need to keep going?

ME AND MY BODY

I'm hungry!

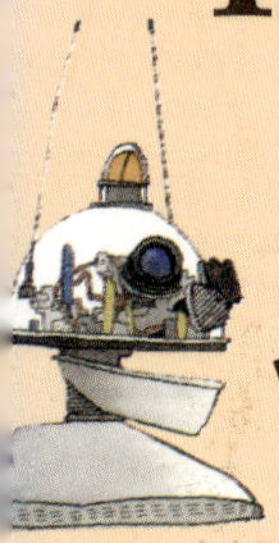

> I have never had a meal in my life. I just don't need food. For me a change of batteries is enough. But it's obvious that you need food and I want to know exactly why.

Starchy foods, like bread and potatoes, and foods with sugar in them give you energy.

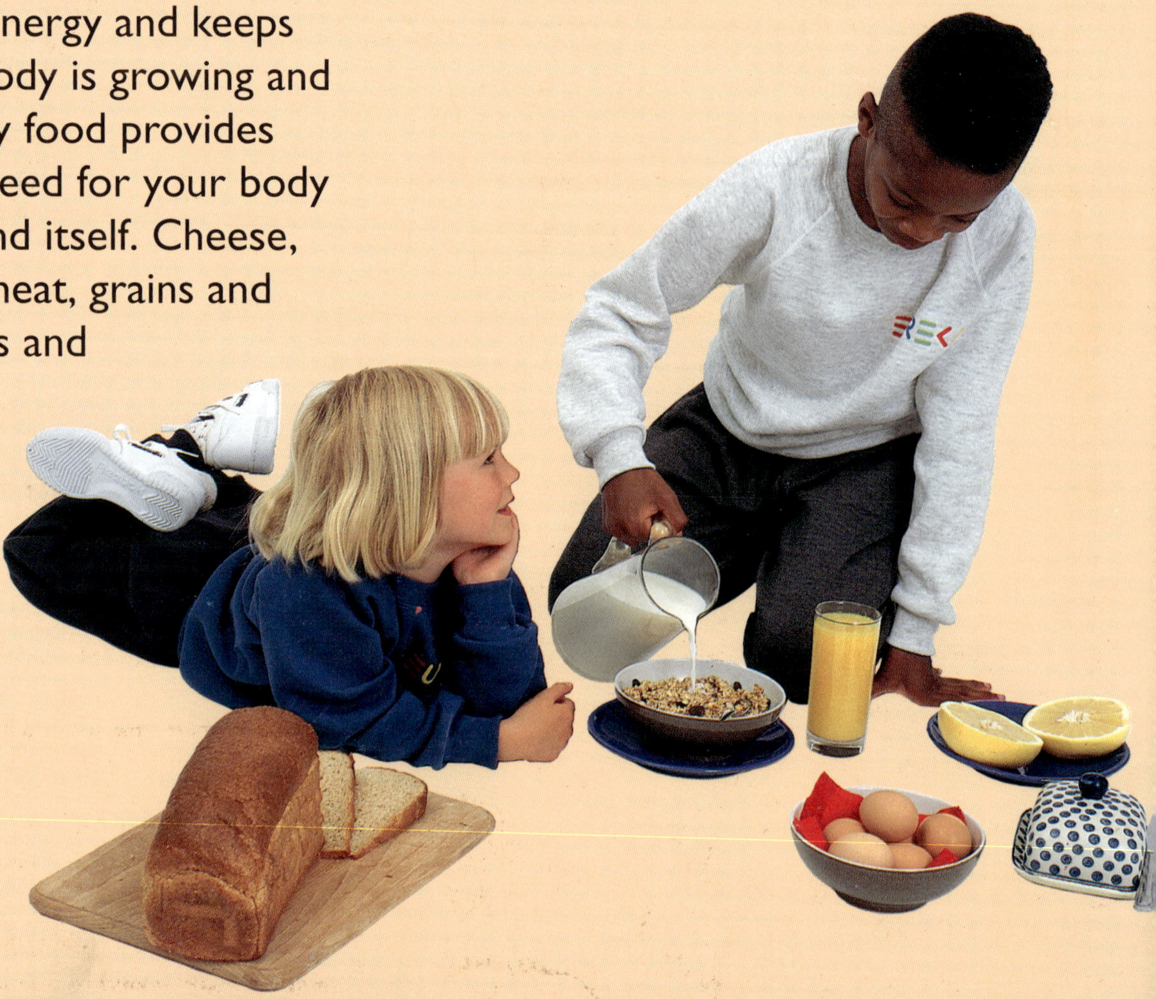

Food gives you energy and keeps you well. Your body is growing and changing. Healthy food provides everything you need for your body to grow and mend itself. Cheese, eggs, milk, fish, meat, grains and pulses (like beans and lentils) are all foods which help muscles and bones to grow.

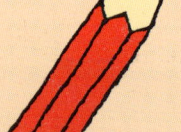

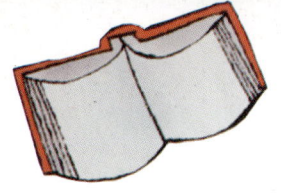

ME AND MY BODY

Different foods help your body in different ways. The vitamins in fruits and vegetables are good for your skin. Brown bread and cereals that contain a lot of fibre keep the stomach and intestines working well. Some foods are less healthy. Too many sugary foods and fatty foods can be harmful to the body, for children and adults. A healthy meal will contain the right balance of all the different types of food.

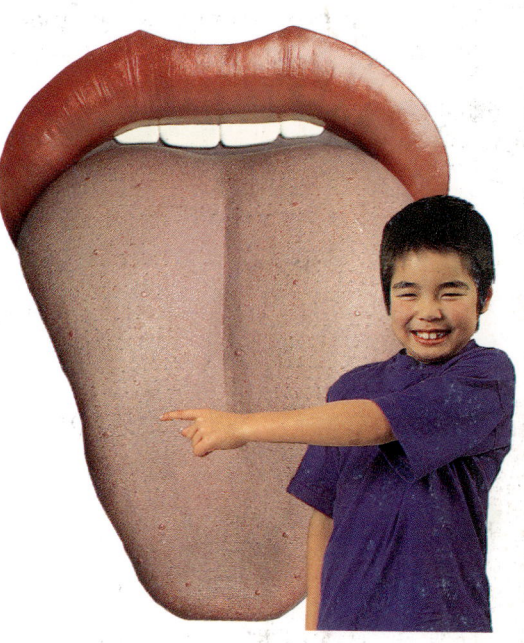

This giant tongue is on display at the EUREKA! Museum. A different area of taste buds lights up depending on which button you press - sweet, sour, salty or bitter.

Scoot investigates

Note it down
Make a list of the foods you like to eat. Put a cross by the ones you think might be less healthy. Now write down why.

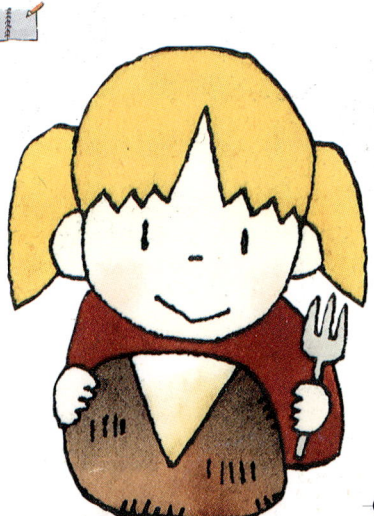

Taste is another one of your senses. Different taste buds on your tongue tell you whether something is sweet or sour, salty or bitter.

Now I know what you like! Remember you have some choice over what to eat. I wonder what would be a healthy balanced meal for a robot - if I needed food ...

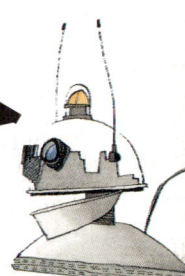

ME AND MY BODY

What happens to the food inside me?

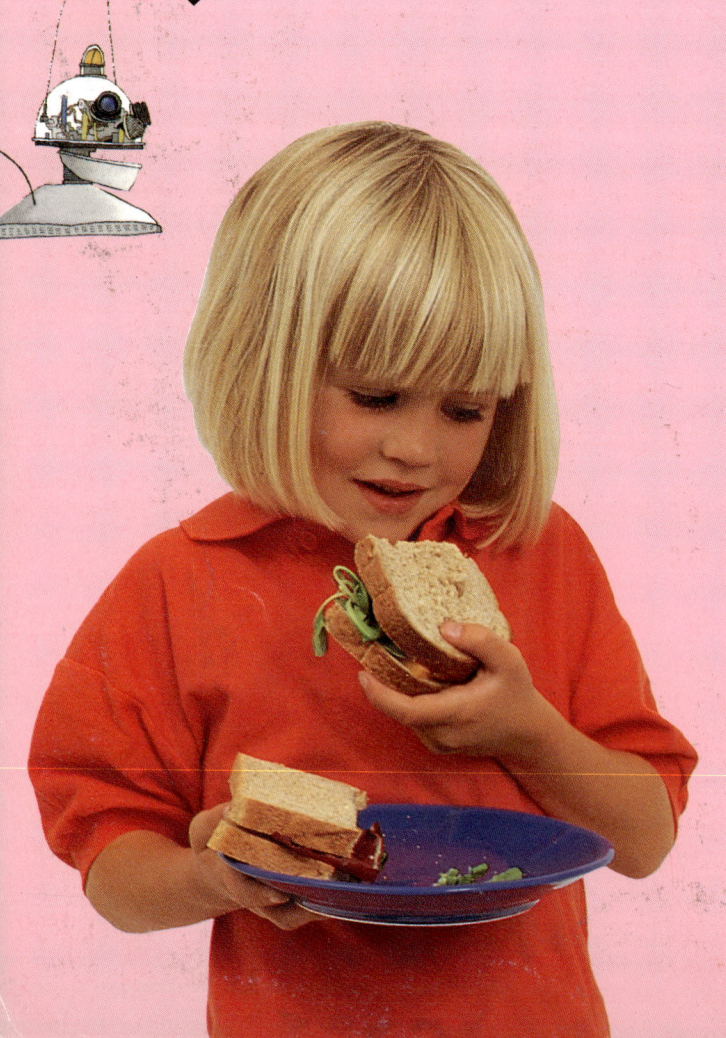

You think about food, you see some food, you take a big bite. And then what? It just disappears and gets mixed up? I think I should find out exactly what goes on down in your tummy.

Sharp front teeth cut up your food into small pieces. Big back teeth crush and mash. Your tongue pushes the food around and mixes in saliva to make it nice and wet.

When you swallow, the food is pushed down the back of your throat into the stomach. Here it is churned up and becomes even more liquid. The soupy food then passes from the stomach into a long tube called the intestine. More juices are mixed in until the food is completely digested. The goodness is passed into your bloodstream to be taken round your body. The waste that your body doesn't want finally comes out through the opening at the bottom of the intestine when you go to the toilet.

Scoot investigates

Experiment
The human intestine is nine metres long. You can see what that looks like by measuring nine metres of string and stretching it along the floor.

Write
Listen to the noises your tummy makes when you are hungry. Write a poem about them.

> That sounds like a big mess. But now at least I know what happens to your food. Does your body always work so well?

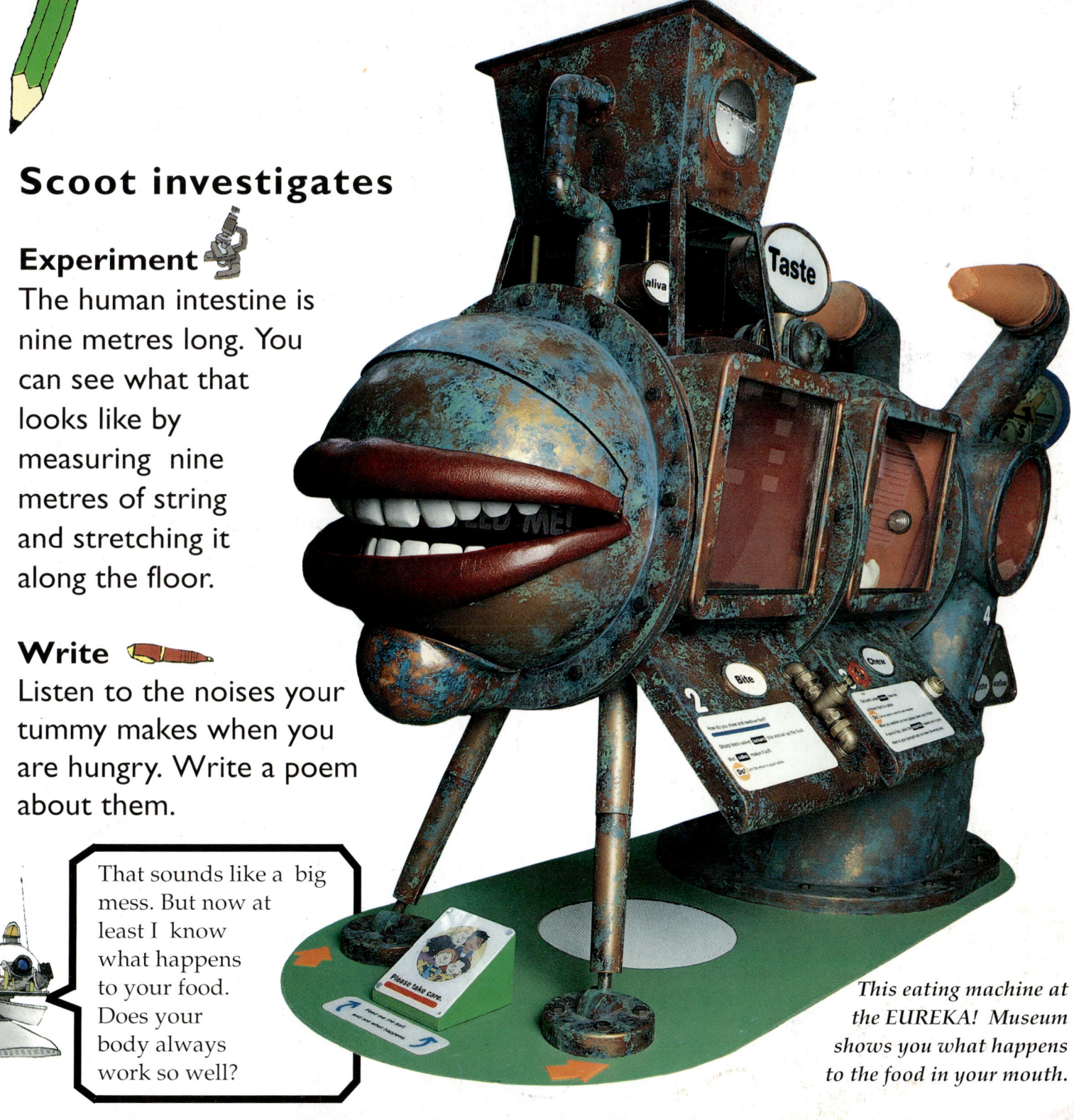

This eating machine at the EUREKA! Museum shows you what happens to the food in your mouth.

ME AND MY BODY

Getting better

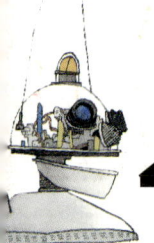

When I break down I have to go to the repair shop. What does your body do when things go wrong? And how do you help it get better?

Healthy food, exercise and sleep all help to keep you well. So what makes you ill?

Sometimes harmful germs get inside your body. You might breathe them in, or cut yourself or eat food that has gone bad.

Then your body's defences have to fight the germs. You might feel hot or achey for a while, but if you keep warm, drink plenty and rest, your body will usually win the battle and get better. Sometimes medicines can help to stop a headache and bring down your temperature, or the doctor might give you antibiotics to kill the harmful germs. People who are seriously hurt or ill need special care from doctors and nurses in hospital.

ME AND MY BODY

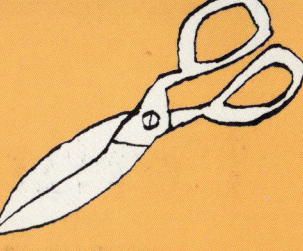

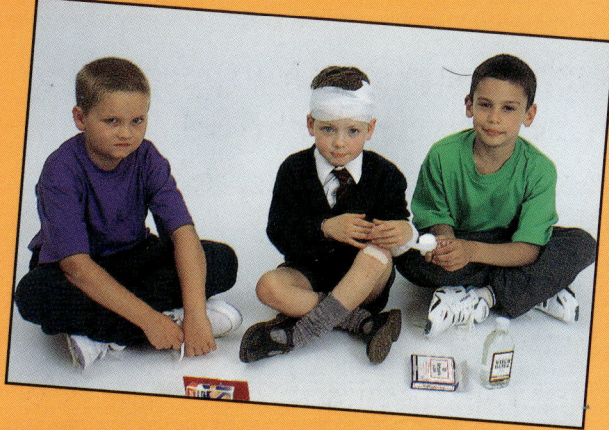

Scoot investigates

Note it down
Write down the illnesses and accidents you have had. Try to remember what they were like, and how quickly you got better. Show your list to a friend and compare your experiences.

Draw
Make a picture showing how you feel when you get ill. Make another showing how you feel when you get better.

> I suppose that with such an amazing body you would get ill sometimes. If I were you I think I would want to look after it very carefully.

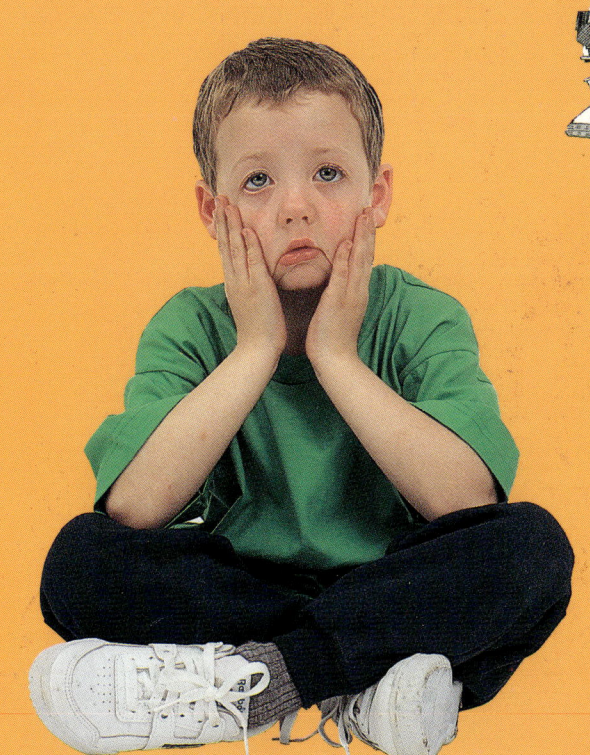

ME AND MY BODY

I'm getting older

> I wonder how old I am? It's quite hard to tell with me. My body never changes from one year to the next. Sometimes I see a bit of rust or flaking paint. But no one could say I'm growing! Now I want to know how you grow. What changes happen? Why grow up anyway?

It's hard to remember a time when you were very small and couldn't do all the things you can do now. You have learned so much since you were a baby. Toddlers who can't run very fast or talk clearly sometimes find life frustrating. But as you get older you can do things better. By the time most children go to school they can walk and talk, feed themselves and use the toilet. They have learned a little about sharing with others and looking after themselves. At school they start to find out about words and numbers, pictures, music and sport.

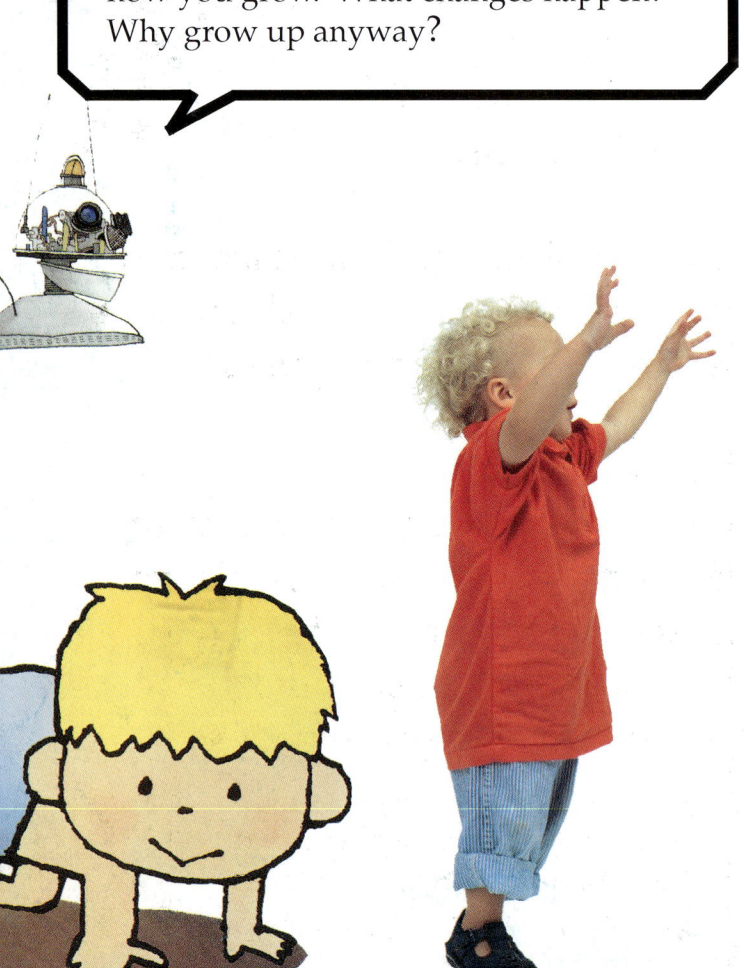

ME AND 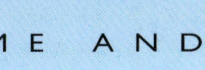 MY BODY

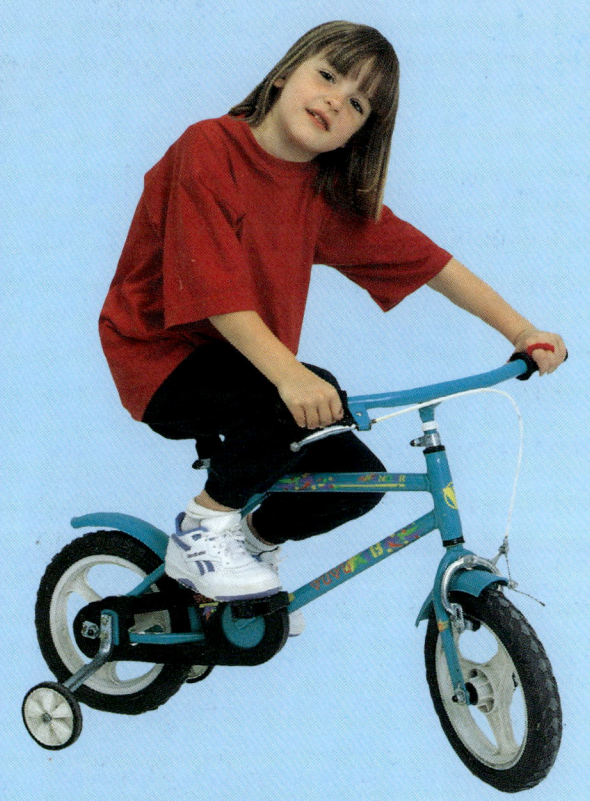

Scoot investigates

Note it down
At what ages did the people in your family learn to walk? Talk? Read? Drive?

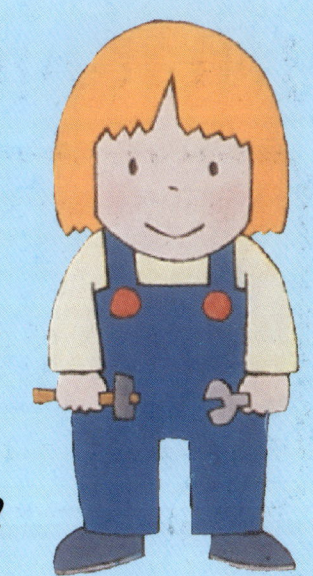

List the skills you have learned in the past year. Can you tell the time, whistle, or swim ten metres?

Draw
Draw yourself as the star of your favourite activity: for example, as a tennis player at Wimbledon, the lead singer of a rock band, etc.

Children learn to do things when they are ready.
For example, some children can tie their laces or ride a bike long before they can read or play the recorder. Others are quite the opposite. The important thing to remember is that you will probably learn to do these things sooner or later if you want to!

I can see that you are getting older and cleverer all the time. But when do children turn into grown-ups? What happens then?

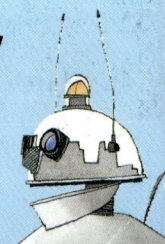

ME AND MY BODY

What happens when I grow up?

> I don't change at all, but over the years I have seen children change into grown-ups and have children of their own. I'd like to know a bit more about these special changes in your bodies.

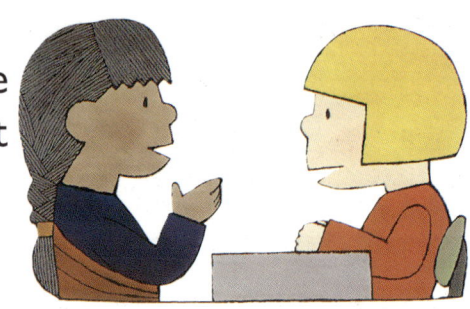

Boys and girls start to change into men and women some time between the ages of eight and fifteen. This stage is called puberty. The changes prepare your bodies to produce babies yourselves when you get older, if that is what you want.

A boy's penis and testicles grow larger. The testicles begin to make sperm. A girl grows breasts and her ovaries start to release an egg cell once a month.

A new life begins the moment a sperm cell from the father fertilises the egg cell inside the mother's womb. The baby grows in the womb inside the mother's tummy. After three months it is still only

The unborn baby is called a foetus. The four-month-old foetus measures fifteen centimetres. This is how it looks inside the mother's womb.

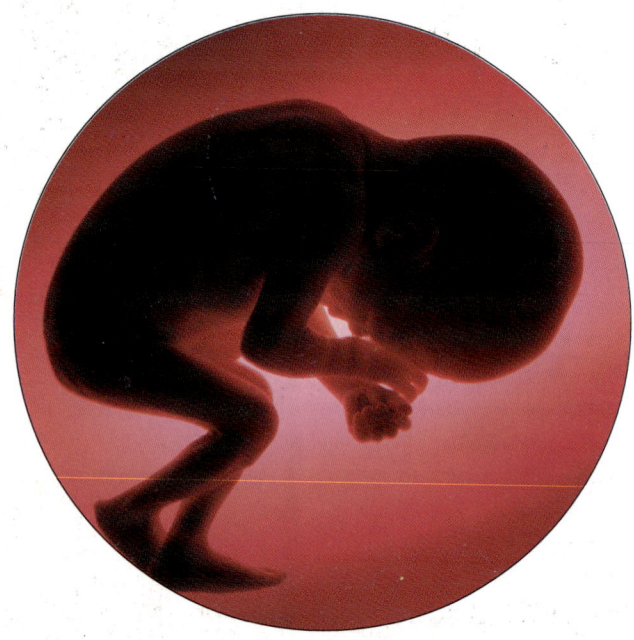

ME AND MY BODY

eight centimetres long but it already looks like a human being and can even suck its thumb! At five and a half months the tiny baby is fully formed. The baby carries on growing until at last after nine months it is ready to be born. Then the mother's muscles push it down the passage from her womb and out into the world. The rest of the family see the new arrival for the first time.

Scoot investigates

Note it down
Stick a photo of yourself as a baby in your book. Talk about what you were like when you were a baby.

Draw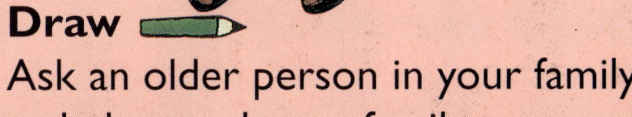
Ask an older person in your family to help you draw a family tree.

> Your bodies are really quite fantastic. Now I want to find out a bit more about what goes on in your heads.

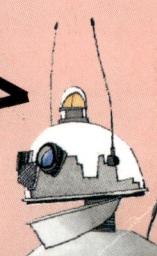

ME AND MY BODY

My dreams

I've never had a dream in my life. When I get turned off at night all my brain waves stop. And during the day I cannot dream either. I can only think about the people in front of me. So how can you dream up people and things that aren't real?

When you dream, your imagination is at work. No one knows why you dream at night. Dreams might be the brain's way of sorting out all the things which have been happening in the day. Even scary dreams may help us to understand ourselves better.

When you are awake you use your imagination to make up stories. You also use it when you listen to stories or music. Your dreams are a very important part of you that no one can take away.

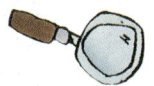 ME AND MY BODY

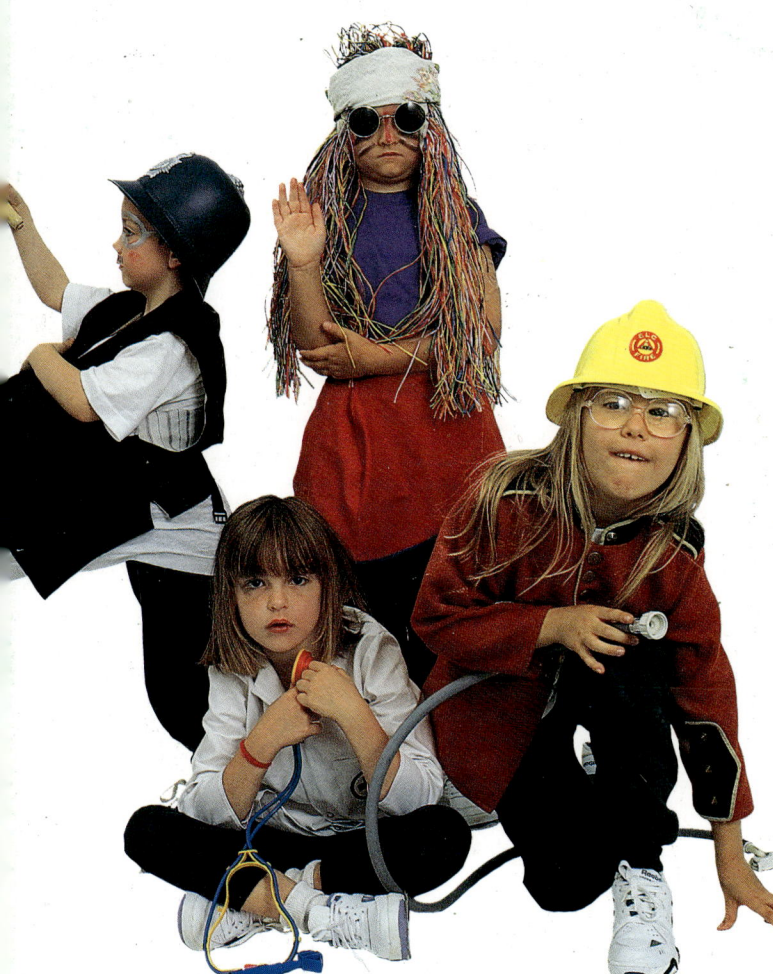

Scoot investigates

Note it down
Make a list of stories you like by authors who have lots of imagination.

Draw
Draw a picture and write about your favourite dream.

Talk
Talk to your friends about what they want to be when they grow up.

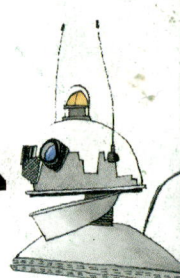

And now, goodbye. I have to go away and think about everything I have learned. I wish I was as clever as you, and could play and dream.

Scoot understands how you can enjoy a daydream about the past. What is more surprising is the way you can imagine the future! In your imagination you can pretend to be anyone.

INDEX

A
accident 22, 23

B
baby 26, 27
bloodstream 16, 17, 18
bones 12, 13, 18
brain 12, 13
breasts 26
breathing 16

D
dreams 28, 29

E
egg cell 26
emotions 10
eyesight 12, 13

F
family tree 27
feelings 10, 11
foetus 26
food 18, 19

G
germs 14, 21
growing 8, 9, 18

H
hearing 13
heart 17
height 8, 9
hospital 22

I
illness 22, 23
imagination 28, 29
intestines 19, 20, 21

L
learning 24, 25
lungs 16

M
muscles 12, 13, 18

O
ovaries 26
oxygen 16, 17

P
penis 26
puberty 26
pulse 17

S
senses 12, 13
skeletons 12, 13
skills 24, 25
skin 14, 15, 19
sperm 26
stomach 19, 20, 21

T
taste 19
taste buds 19
teeth 20
testicles 26
touch 15

W
weight 8, 9
womb 26